Vegan Diet

Simple Vegetarian Cookbook for Beginners

(Delicious and Satisfying Vegan Recipes for Weight Loss)

Brad Cox

Published by Robert Satterfield Publishing House

Vegan Diet Recipes: Simple Vegetarian Cookbook for Beginners (Delicious and Satisfying Vegan Recipes for Weight Loss)

ISBN 978-1-989682-97-5

Legal & Disclaimer

TABLE OF CONTENT

Part 1

Introduction

Year after year, thousands of people both young and old all over the world are embracing vegan lifestyle. As more minds open to this way of life and taste buds welcome the rich tastes of natural foods, being vegan is getting less lonely and variety of recipes are being developed to cater for divers tastes.

If you are just starting out, the variety of recipes and sometimes conflicting voices on what is delicious or not may be a little frustrating. Relax, don't get so caught up on what food tastes better or not, your taste buds are very flexible-they'll adapt to the new tastes and you'll find yourself enjoying foods you never thought you would eat.

Having a catalog of recipes or volumes upon volumes of cookbooks will not guarantee you a plate of delicious meal on the dinner table. You'll have to roll up your sleeves and work the saucepans. However, cooking doesn't have to be one more thing on your "stress-list." Preparing plant based meals can be simple, fun, and delicious.

After a busy day, you don't want to get home and work yourself crazy just to get dinner on the table. This book will make it possible for you to make something hearty no matter how tired or lazy you are. It is a collection of simple 5-ingredient recipes your taste buds will gladly welcome. You'll be able to put together these soups, salads, and smoothies in a few minutes with less effort and without much fuss.

If you are new to this way of eating, don't worry! Vegan meals are not dull or tasteless as most people assume. You'll discover a couple of delicious and healthy meals you'll come to enjoy and even fall in love with. Just start simply, may be with a glass of breakfast smoothie and then gradually move to salads and stews, or more complicated recipes.

I wrote this book to share some of my favorite recipes that are simple to make. If you are looking for something complicated, you may be disappointed.

But if you are searching for easy yet delicious smoothies, soups, and salads, this book was written with you in mind.

Brace yourself for a delicious journey!

Tomato Soup

Serves: 2

Prep: 5 minutes

Cook: 30 minutes

Ingredients

- 6 large tomatoes, cored
- 1 onion
- 2 garlic cloves
- 2 cups coconut milk
- 1/3 cup noni
- Salt and pepper

Preparation

- Add tomatoes, onions, garlic, and coconut milk in a blender.
- Blend until smooth.
- Pour puree into a pot and cook for approximately 25 minutes.

- Add noni juice, mix well.
- Taste and season with salt and pepper. Enjoy!

Miso Soup

Serves: 2

Prep: 5 minutes

Cook: 5 minutes

Ingredients

- 2 scallions, chopped
- 4 ounces tofu, chopped
- 3 cups water
- 1 cup mixed vegetables
- 1 tablespoons mellow white miso

Preparation

- In a pot, add water, tofu, and vegetables.
- Place over high heat and bring to the boil.
- Turn heat to medium and let it cook for 3 minutes.

- Meanwhile, add miso and water (2 tablespoons) in a small bowl. Stir until dissolved.
- Add the mixture into the soup. Mix well and serve.
- Top each serving with chopped scallion.

Traditional Miso Soup

Serves: 4

Prep: 5 minutes

Cook: 5 minutes

Ingredients

- 6 (3 inches each) kombu pieces
- 3 scallions (green parts), sliced
- 32 ounces container vegetable broth
- 12.3 ounces container extra firm tofu
- 4 tablespoons miso
- Freshly ground black pepper

Preparation

- In a pot, add kombu and broth. Put to simmer over medium heat.

- Add tofu and continue simmering for a few minutes.
- Meanwhile, dissolve 4 tablespoons of miso in water and pour into the soup. Mix well.
- Add scallions and season to taste with pepper. Enjoy!

Cauliflower Soup

Serves: 4

Prep: 5 minutes

Cook: 17 minutes

Ingredients

- ½ head cauliflower, chopped
- 4 garlic cloves, chopped
- 1 yellow onion, chopped
- 2 cups vegetable broth
- 1 tablespoon rosemary, fresh, chopped
- 1 tablespoon olive oil

Preparation

- In a pot, add olive oil and heat over medium heat. Cook onions until tender, about 5 minutes. Add garlic and cook for 1 minute, stirring from time to time.

- Add rosemary and cauliflower. Cook for 5 minutes.
- Add vegetable broth and bring to a boil over high heat.
- Lower heat to a gentle simmer. Let simmer for 5 minutes.
- Blend until smooth. Enjoy!

Potato and Leek Soup

Serves: 8

Prep: 10 minutes

Cook: 25 minutes

Ingredients

- ¾ pounds leek, chopped
- 1.1 pounds new potatoes, peeled, quartered
- 2 minced garlic clove
- 1 teaspoon salt
- 4 cups water

Preparation

- In a pot, add leek, potatoes, garlic, salt and water.
- Cook until potatoes are tender.
- Blend until smooth and serve.

Black Bean Soup

Serves: 4

Prep: 5 minutes

Cook: 15 minutes

Ingredients

- 2 (15 ounces each) cans drained black beans
- 1 cup vegetable broth
- 1 teaspoon chili powder
- 1 teaspoon cumin
- 16 ounces salsa

Preparation

- Add salsa, chili powder, cumin, vegetable broth, and 1 can of black beans in a soup pot.
- Bring the mixture to a boil.

- Reduce heat and simmer for 10 minutes.
- Stir from time to time as it simmers.
- Let cool and blend until smooth.
- Add reserved beans and cook for 5 minutes.
- Taste and season as desired.
- Enjoy!

Pea and Mint Soup

Serves: 4

Prep: 5 minutes

Cook: 25 minutes

Ingredients

- 500g pea, frozen
- 350g baking potato, peeled, cut into cubes
- 1 tablespoon mint, fresh
- 1 white scallion
- 3 ¼ cups vegetable stock
- 1 tablespoon olive oil
- Salt and pepper

Preparation

- In a soup pot, add olive oil and heat over medium.
- When hot, add onions and cook for 2 minutes.
- Add potatoes and cook for 5 minutes, stirring occasionally.
- Pour in stock and put to simmer until potatoes are tender, about 15 minutes.
- Mix in peas and continue simmering for 5 minutes.
- Add mint and heat through.
- If you like it smooth, blend before serving.

Spring Vegetable Soup

Serves: 5

Prep: 10 minutes

Cook: 30 minutes

Ingredients

- 2 large potatoes, peeled, diced
- 3 medium carrots, peeled, diced
- 1 onion, peeled, sliced

- 3 celery stalks, sliced
- 2 tablespoons sunflower oil
- 1 cup peas, fresh
- 1 vegetable stock cube
- Salt, to taste

Preparation

- Add oil in a soup pot and heat over medium-high. Add onions and cook for 4 minutes or until tender.
- Add potatoes, peas, carrots, and celery. Continue cooking for 2 minutes.
- Add water and salt. Bring the mixture to a boil.
- Lower heat and add vegetable stock cube.
- Cook until potatoes are tender, about 30 minutes.

Potato Black Bean Chili

Serves: 6

Prep: 10 minutes

Cook: 45 minutes

Ingredients

- 3 sweet potatoes, diced

- 1 (15 ounces) can black beans
- 1 (16 ounces) jar salsa
- 2 cups vegetable stock
- 2 cups water
- 1 white onion, chopped
- Salt and pepper

Preparation

- Add oil in a pot and heat over medium.
- When hot, add onions and cook until tender.
- Add potatoes and cook for 3 minutes.
- Add all remaining ingredients except beans.
- Bring to a boil. Reduce heat to a gentle simmer.
- Mix in beans, cover, and continue cooking until potatoes soften, about 20 minutes.
- Taste and season as desired.
- Serve with your favorite topping.

Fruit Smoothie

Serves: 1

Prep: 5 minutes

Ingredients

- 1/3 cup dragon fruit, frozen
- 4 bananas, frozen
- 1 teaspoon coconut nectar
- ½ cup water

Preparation

- In a blender, add banana, coconut nectar, dragon fruit, and water. Blend until smooth.

Berry Smoothie

Serves: 2

Prep: 5 minutes

Ingredients

- 1 cup berries, frozen
- 1 cup fruit juice, fresh
- ½ cup banana, frozen
- 1 cup spinach
- 1 tablespoon flaxseed meal

Preparation

- In the blender, add berries, banana, spinach, juice, and flaxseed meal.
- Blend until smooth. Enjoy!

Green Smoothie

Serves: 1

Prep: 5 minutes

Ingredients

- 2 handfuls spinach
- 2 bananas
- 2 cups almond milk
- 2 tablespoons almond butter

Preparation

- In the blender, add banana, spinach, almond butter, and almond milk.
- Blend until smooth.
- Enjoy!

Avocado Smoothie

Serves: 1

Prep: 5 minutes

Ingredients

- 1 avocado, peeled, pits removed
- 1 cup almond milk
- ½ banana
- 5 ice cubes

Preparation

- In the blender, add all ingredients and blend until smooth.
- Enjoy!

Tropical Smoothie

Serves: 2

Prep: 5 minutes

Ingredients

- 1 cup pineapple chunks, frozen
- 1 cup mango chunks, frozen
- 1 banana, peeled
- 1 orange, peeled, sliced
- 1 cup coconut water

Preparation

- In the blender, add orange, pineapple, mango, banana, and coconut water.
- Blend until smooth. Enjoy!

Breakfast Smoothie

Serves: 1

Prep: 5 minutes

Ingredients

- 2 tablespoon chia seeds
- 1 tablespoon coconut oil
- 1 cup almond milk
- 1 cup fruit juice, fresh
- 1 banana
- 1 teaspoon ginger

Preparation

- In the blender, add all ingredients and blend until smooth. Enjoy!

Berry Quinoa Smoothie

Serves: 2

Prep: 5 minutes

Ingredients

- ½ cup quinoa, cooked
- 1 cup mixed berries, frozen
- ½ cup almond milk
- 1 banana
- 2 tablespoons peanut butter

Preparation

- In the blender, add quinoa, banana, berries, almond milk, and peanut butter.
- Blend until smooth. Enjoy!

Beet Fruit Smoothie

Serves: 1

Prep: 5 minutes

Ingredients

- 1 green apple, cored
- 1 raw red beet, peeled
- 1/3 cup fresh pomegranate juice
- 2 oranges, peeled
- 1 cup ice, crushed

Preparation

- In the blender, add apple, beet, oranges, ice, and pomegranate juice.
- Blend until smooth. Enjoy!

Berry Smoothie

Serves: 2

Prep: 5 minutes

Ingredients

- 1 cup raspberries, frozen
- 1 cup strawberries, frozen
- 1 cup blueberries, frozen
- 2 bananas
- 1 cup almond milk, unsweetened

Preparation

- In the blender, add all ingredients and blend until smooth.

Mexican Quinoa

Serves: 4

Prep: 5 minutes

Cook: 10 minutes

Ingredients

- 1 cup corn kernels, fresh
- 3 cups white quinoa, cooked
- 1 cup salsa
- 1 tablespoon cumin, ground
- 15 ounces can black beans

Preparation

- Place a skillet over medium heat. Cook beans and corn for 3 minutes or until corn softens.
- Mix in cumin and quinoa. Continue cooking for 3 minutes, stir often.
- Add salsa and cook for an additional 2 minutes, stirring occasionally.
- Let it cool and serve.

Watermelon Mint Salad

Serves: 4

Prep: 5 minutes

Ingredients

- 5 mint leaves, chopped

- 8 large watermelon cubes, cut into small cubes

Preparation

- In a large bowl, mix together watermelon and mint leaves.
- Toss and serve.

Tomato Bean Salad

Serves: 2

Prep: 15 minutes

Ingredients

- 250g sundried tomatoes
- 2 (400g each) cans cannellini beans, drained and rinsed
- Fresh juice and zest from 1 lemon
- 100g watercress

Preparation

- Toss together all ingredients in a large bowl.
- Serve and enjoy!

Part 2

Introduction

This vegan baking and dessert cookbook includes a variety of unique and delicious cake, cookie and bread recipes that you can easily make at home. As a professional vegan baker I have come across all kinds of vegan baking recipes, and I would like to share my favorite vegan baking recipes with you. I have provided easy to follow steps in these recipes, so both beginner and novice vegan bakers can make these recipes.

These recipes were the most popular in my bakery, and I think you will really enjoy them!

Chapter 1: Vegan Bread And Muffin Recipes

Oatmeal Brown Bread

Ingredients

2-1/2 cups course whole wheat flour

1 cup oatmeal

3/4 cup wheat germ

2 teaspoons sugar

2 teaspoons baking powder

1 1/2 teaspoons salt

1 teaspoon baking soda

1 1/2 cups soy milk

Egg substitute (2 egg equivalents)

2 tablespoon olive oil

Directions

In a medium bowl, mix all the dry ingredients - flour, oatmeal, wheat germ, sugar, baking powder, salt, and baking soda. Create a well in the middle of the dry ingredients.

In the well, add the milk, eggs, and olive oil; mix the batter well. If the mix is too thick, add a little more milk if necessary.

In a greased bread pan, add the batter and smooth the top. Make two diagonal cuts on the top of the bread.

Bake in the oven at 425 degrees F for 15 minutes. Reduce the heat to 375 F and bake for another 40 minutes.

Take out of the oven and test to see if done. To test if the bread is done, either tap the bottom and listen for a hollow sound or insert a skewer into the middle of the loaf and check if it comes out clean.

If not, bake for another few minutes and re-check.

Zucchini Chocolate Bread

Ingredients

5 tablespoons ground flax + 10 tablespoons water

3 cups flour

1/4 cup cocoa powder

1 tablespoon cinnamon

1 teaspoon baking soda

1/2 teaspoon baking powder

1 teaspoon salt

2 cups sugar

1 cup vegetable oil

2/3 cup soy milk

1 teaspoon vanilla

2 cups zucchini, shredded

1 cup vegan semi-sweet chocolate chips

1 cup walnuts, chopped, optional

Directions

Preheat oven to 350 F. Spray two 9x5 inch loaf pans with nonstick spray. For flax eggs, microwave flax meal and water for 30 seconds, stir, microwave, 30 more seconds, and stir again.

Combine all dry ingredients in a large bowl and mix well. Add vegetable oil, and use a fork to stir. It will be dry but stir as well as possible. Then add the flax eggs. Continue to mix.

Add milk and vanilla, and stir until well blended. Add zucchini, chocolate chips and walnuts, if using, and blend them in. The mixture should be nice and smooth; moist looking.

Spoon into prepared loaf pans. Bake 55-60 minutes. Cool in pans for 10 minutes, then remove and cool completely.

Chocolate Chip Pumpkin Muffins

Ingredients

3/4 cup sugar

1/4 cup canola oil

egg substitutes (2 egg equivalent), prepared

3/4 cup canned pumpkin

1/4 cup water

1-1/2 cups flour

3/4 teaspoon baking powder

1/2 teaspoon baking soda

1/2 teaspoon ground cinnamon

1/4 teaspoon salt

1/2 cup vegan chocolate chips

Directions

Preheat the oven to 400 degrees F. Grease and flour muffin pan or use paper liners.

In a bowl, mix sugar, oil, and egg replacer. Add pumpkin and water.

In separate bowl, mix flour, baking powder, baking soda, cinnamon, and salt. Add the wet mixture and stir in chocolate chips.

Fill muffin cups 2/3 full with batter and bake for 20 to 25 minutes.

Applesauce Muffins

Ingredients

1 cup whole wheat flour

1 cup oatmeal

2 teaspoon baking powder

1 teaspoon cinnamon

few dashes ground cloves

1/2 cup chopped walnuts

1/2 cup raisins

egg substitute (2 eggs equivalent)

3/4 cup applesauce

Directions

Mix dry ingredients. Add applesauce and stir until consistency is good, then add prepared egg replacer and mix again.

Transfer to muffin tins (nonstick) and bake at 375F for 25 minutes or until tests done.

Zucchini Blueberry Muffins

Ingredients

1 3/4 cups of flour

2 teaspoons of baking powder

1/2 of a teaspoon of allspice

1/4 of a teaspoon of salt

1/3 of a cup of sugar

1 teaspoon of vanilla extract

1/2 of a banana, mashed

3/4 of a cup of pureed zucchini

1/4 of a cup of unsweetened applesauce

1 cup of fresh blueberries

1 tablespoon of water

Directions

Combine dry and wet ingredients separately. Mix them together, and fold in the blueberries.

Spoon into a muffin pan sprayed with cooking spray and bake at 400 F for 15 minutes.

Whole Grain Bread

Ingredients

1 cup water

1/3 cup vanilla soy milk

1 1/2 tablespoons margarine

1/3 cup blackstrap molasses

1 1/2 cups whole wheat flour

1 1/2 cups rolled oats

1/2 cup white flour

1 teaspoon salt

1 dash cinnamon

1/4 cup sunflower seeds

1/2 teaspoon orange rind

1 1/2 teaspoons active dry yeast

Directions

Place all ingredients in the bread machine in the order instructed by the manufacturer. Select the basic setting with a light crust.

Banana Walnut Bread

Ingredients

2 cups raw zucchini, shredded

3/4 cup mashed banana

1 cup sugar

3 tbsp ground flax seed + 8 tbsp water (egg replacement)

2 tablespoons vegetable oil

3 teaspoons vanilla

3 cups flour

1 teaspoon salt

1 teaspoon baking powder

3 teaspoons cinnamon

1/3 cup chopped walnuts

Directions

Preheat oven to 325 degrees. Oil two 9" x 5" x 3" loaf pans or spray with cooking spray.

In a small bowl, whisk ground flax with water. In a large bowl, combine flour, salt, baking powder and cinnamon.

Add flax mixture, zucchini, sugar, banana, oil, and vanilla. Mix until just combined. Fold in walnuts.

Pour half the mixture into each pan. Bake for about 1 hour, or until toothpick in center comes out clean.

Whole Wheat Raisin Bread

Ingredients

6 cups whole wheat flour

1/3 cup brown sugar

1 tablespoon salt

5 teaspoons dry yeast

3 1/4 cups warm water

2/3 cups raisins or dates

Directions

In a large bowl mix all the dry ingredients together. Add the water and beat the mixture to make a nice thick batter.

Pour it into 2 greased loaf pans and smooth out the tops. Cover the pans with greased plastic wrap and let it rise until doubled in volume. Bake at 400F for about 45 minutes or until a tooth pick comes out clean.

Orange Raspberry Muffins

Ingredients

7 1/2 tablespoons water

3 tablespoons flaxseed meal

1/3 cup frozen raspberries, crumbled

1/2 cup maple syrup

1/3 orange, zested and juiced

3 tablespoons coconut oil, melted

1 teaspoon vanilla extract

2/3 cup gluten-free all-purpose baking mix

2/3 cup gluten-free oat flour

1 teaspoon baking soda

1 teaspoon baking powder

1 teaspoon xanthan gum

1/4 teaspoon salt

cooking spray

Directions

Preheat oven to 350 degrees F (175 degrees C). Grease a muffin tin with cooking spray.

Whisk water and flaxseed meal together in a small bowl to make flax eggs. Let stand until thickened, about 5 minutes.

Place raspberries in a microwave-safe bowl. Heat in the microwave until thawed, 10 to 15 seconds. Stir in flax eggs, maple syrup, orange zest, orange juice, coconut oil, and vanilla extract.

Whisk baking mix, oat flour, baking soda, baking powder, xanthan gum, and salt together in a bowl. Add raspberry mixture; mix quickly with a spatula until batter is combined.

Scoop batter into the muffin tin, filling each cup 3/4 full. Bake in the preheated oven until browned, about 15 minutes.

Cranberry Muffins

Ingredients

2 cups flour

1 cup ground walnuts

1/4 cup sugar

4 teaspoons baking powder

1/4 teaspoon cinnamon

1/4 teaspoon nutmeg

1-1/2 cups non-dairy milk, with vanilla

2 egg replacers, prepared

1/3 cup olive oil

1 teaspoon grated lemon rind

a squeeze of juice from grated lemon (optional)

3 cups vegan bran flakes

1 cup cranberries, fresh or frozen or dried

Pinch of salt

Directions

Preheat oven to 400 F. Lightly grease muffin tin.

In a bowl, mix together dry ingredients except for branflakes.

In another bowl, mix together wet ingredients. Fold bran flakes into wet ingredients. Let stand for a few minutes.

Add wet ingredients to dry ingredients, stirring until just moistened. Fold in whole cranberries.

Bake at 400 F. for 23 to 25 minutes.

Apple Cinnamon Muffins

Ingredients

1/2 cup unbleached flour

3/4 cup whole wheat flour

1 1/2 teaspoon cinnamon

1 teaspoon baking powder

1/2 teaspoon baking soda

1 cup soy milk

1 packet of regular instant oatmeal

1/2 cup oat bran

1/4 cup maple sugar crystals (or brown sugar substitute)

2 tablespoons canola oil

1/4 cup unsweetened apple sauce

1 1/2 cups shopped or shredded peeled apples

Directions

Coat 12 muffin cups with nonstick spray and set aside. Preheat oven at 350F.

In medium bowl combine flours, cinnamon, baking powder and, baking soda.

Peel apples. You can either finely chop them or shred them with a grater. In a large bowl beat together the soy milk, oatmeal, oat bran, maple crystals, oil, and applesauce.

Add flour mixture, medium bowl, to liquid mixture. Careful not to over mix. Fold in apples, spoon batter into muffin cups and bake at 400F for 20 minutes. Use a toothpick to test doneness.

Remove muffins, let cool for 5 minutes.

Banana Coconut Muffins

Ingredients

1/2 cup of oats

1 cup all purpose flour

1/2 cup whole wheat flour

1 1/2 teaspoons baking powder

1/2 teaspoon baking soda

1 1/2 teaspoons cinnamon

1 1/2 cups mashed ripe bananas

1 cup sugar

7/8 cup of cooking oil

1/4 cup coconut milk

3/4 cup shredded coconut (sweetened)

1 teaspoon vanilla extract

Egg replacer equivalent to 2 eggs

Directions

Preheat oven 350F. Grind the oats up so they are pretty fine but they can have a few whole oats.

Put all the dry ingredients (except sugar) in a medium size bowl. In another bowl, mix all the wet ingredients and the sugar together.

Mix the wet and dry ingredients together. Lightly grease a muffin tray and fill each dip about 3/4 of the way with the mixture.

Place in the oven for 25-30 minutes.

Strawberry Muffins

Ingredients

3 tablespoons powdered egg replacer

1/4 cup water

1 cup evaporated cane sugar

1 cup whole wheat flour

1 teaspoon baking soda

1 – 6 ounce container blueberry flavored coconut milk yogurt

1 tablespoon vanilla

1 tablespoon almond milk

6 sliced strawberries

1 cup blueberry granola

Directions

Preheat oven to 350 F. Prepare a muffin pan with 8 liners.

Mix together water and egg replacer in a small bowl. In a large bowl, combine sugar, flour and baking soda. In a separate bowl, combine yogurt, vanilla, and almond milk. Add all wet ingredients to dry bowl and stir until just mixed and then gently stir in the strawberries.

Divide batter between 8 cupcake liners. Top each muffin with blueberry granola. Bake for 22 minutes or until done.

Carrot Apple Muffins

Ingredients

2 1/2 tablespoons ground flax seed

7 tablespoons hot water

1/3 cup canola oil

2/3 cup nondairy milk

2 teaspoons vanilla extract

2/3 cup packed brown sugar

2 cups carrot, peeled and shredded

1 large apple, unpeeled and shredded

1/2 cup raisins

1/2 cup dried coconut flakes

1/2 cup walnuts

1 cup all-purpose flour

1 cup whole wheat flour

2 teaspoons baking soda

2 teaspoons cinnamon

1/2 teaspoon salt

Directions

Preheat oven to 350 F and line a muffin pan. In a small bowl, whisk together flax seed and hot water to make an egg replacer. Set aside.

Pulse the carrots and apple together in a food processor until chopped into very fine pieces, but not pureed.

In a large mixing bowl, mix together wet ingredients, sugar, carrot, and apple. Stir in remaining ingredients, and mix gently until fully incorporated. Try not to over mix.

Spoon into prepared muffin tins. Fill according to how big you want your muffins to be. Bake for 25 minutes. Let cool completely before serving.

Banana Muffins

Ingredients

1 1/2 cups flour

1/3 cup margarine

1/2 cup sugar

1 teaspoon baking soda

1 teaspoon baking powder

1/2 teaspoon salt

3 mashed bananas

Egg substitute (1 egg equivalent)

Directions

Mix all ingredients well in a medium sized bowl. Pour mixture into muffin tins, bake in the oven at 375 F for 20-25 minutes.

Pumpkin Applesauce Muffins

Ingredients

2 cups all-purpose flour

1 cup brown sugar

1/2 cup white sugar

1/2 cup whole wheat flour

4 teaspoons baking soda

2 teaspoons ground cinnamon

2 teaspoons ground allspice

2 teaspoons salt

1 teaspoon baking powder

2 cups canned pumpkin puree

2 large apples - peeled, cored, and grated

2 tablespoons dry vegan egg replacer

1 1/4 cups applesauce

1/4 cup vegetable oil

cooking spray

Directions

Preheat oven to 375 degrees F (190 degrees C). Grease 2 muffin tins with cooking spray.

Combine all-purpose flour, brown sugar, white sugar, whole wheat flour, baking soda, cinnamon, allspice, salt, and baking powder in a large bowl. Mix in pumpkin puree and apples.

Pour egg replacer into a bowl. Stir in applesauce gradually to avoid lumps. Whisk in oil. Add to the flour mixture; mix well until batter is smooth.

Spoon batter into the greased muffin cups, filling each one almost to the top.

Bake in the preheated oven until a toothpick inserted into the center comes out clean, about 25 minutes. Cool in the pan for 5 minutes. Transfer to a wire rack to cool completely.

Strawberry Applesauce Muffins

Ingredients

2 cups soy milk

3/4 cup unsweetened applesauce

2 tablespoons white vinegar

4 teaspoons vanilla extract

2 1/2 cups white whole wheat flour

2 cups turbinado sugar

1 cup whole wheat flour

1 cup rolled oats

2 teaspoons baking soda

1 teaspoon salt

1 cup diced strawberries

cooking spray

Directions

Preheat oven to 350 degrees F (175 degrees C). Grease 2 muffin tins with cooking spray.

Mix soy milk, applesauce, vinegar, and vanilla extract together in a bowl.

Sift white whole wheat flour and whole wheat flour together into a separate bowl. Add oats, baking soda, and salt in a separate bowl. Mix in soy milk mixture until smooth. Let batter sit for 5 minutes.

Fold strawberries into the batter. Fill muffin tins 2/3 full of batter.

Bake in the preheated oven until muffin tops are brown and sides pull away from the tin, 30 to 40 minutes.

Lemon Squares

Ingredients

Crust:

1 cup all-purpose flour

5 tablespoons margarine

1/4 cup granulated sugar

Filling:

3 egg replacers

3/4 cup granulated sugar

3 tablespoons all-purpose flour

1 teaspoon real vanilla

1/2 teaspoon baking powder

1/8 teaspoon salt

2 lemons, zested and juiced

powdered sugar, optional

Directions

Preheat oven to 350 degrees F.

To make crust:

In a bowl, combine crust ingredients and press into 8 X 8 inch pan. Bake for 15 minutes.

To make filling:

While crust is baking, beat the egg replacers in a bowl until foamy. Add the remainder of the filling ingredients and mix together. Pour over the crust, and bake 20 minutes, or until set.

Let cool before serving.

Vegan Cheesecake

Ingredients

Crust:

18 vegan graham crackers or other cookies, crumbled

1/2 cup canola oil

1 tablespoon all-purpose flour

1 tablespoon agave or maple syrup

Filling:

1 (10-ounce or 300 g) package silken tofu, pressed lightly to remove water

2/3 cup raw cashews, soaked overnight and drained

1 tablespoon lemon juice

2 teaspoons canola oil

1/3 cup raw sugar or other sweetener

3-1/2 teaspoons Egg Replacer (no water added)

1/2 teaspoon vanilla extract

1/2 teaspoon salt

Directions

To make crust:

Combine all crust ingredients in a large bowl. Mix until well incorporated, and then press into pie dish.

To make filling:

Combine soaked cashews, silken tofu, canola oil, and lemon juice in a blender; pulse until completely smooth and creamy.

Transfer mixture to a bowl and whisk in sugar, egg replacer, vanilla, and salt until completely dissolved, making sure there are no lumps or sugar crystals. Carefully spoon mixture into the crust.

Bake at 375 F for 25 to 30 minutes, until set. Remove from oven and let cool.

Place in fridge for at least five hours to chill.

Vegan Chocolate Fudge Brownies

Ingredients

1/4 cup canola oil

1/3 cup water

1 cup organic sugar

1 cup organic unbleached flour

1 tablespoon ground flax seed

1/3 cup unsweetened cocoa powder

1/2 teaspoon baking powder

1/4 teaspoon salt

Directions

Preheat oven to 350 F. Mix wet ingredients in large bowl, then add in all the dry ingredients and mix. Do not over mix.

Place in oven and bake for 20-25 minutes.

Chocolate Vegan Cheesecake

Ingredients

1 (12 ounce) package silken tofu

1 (8 ounce) tub vegan cream cheese

3/4 cup sugar

1 (12 ounce) package vegan chocolate chips

3 tablespoons maple syrup

1 (9") vegan graham cracker pie crust

Directions

In blender, blend tofu until smooth. With an electric mixer in medium bowl, combine vegan sugar and cream cheese and 2 tablespoons of the smoothed tofu, and beat until smooth.

Add cream cheese mixture to blender with remaining tofu. Blend again until smooth.

Melt chocolate chips in double boiler, or microwave. Add melted chips to blender, blend until chocolate is mixed, this may require some stirring. After chips and mixture are well blended, add maple syrup, blend for 30 seconds.

Pour mixture into pie crust until full, and refrigerate until set.

Apple Cake

Ingredients

1 cup flour

1 cup semolina

1 cup sugar

1 teaspoon baking powder

1 cup vegan margarine, melted

5 large or 8-10 small apples

Directions

Preheat oven to 375F degrees.

Mix flour, sugar, semolina and baking powder in a bowl. Peel and grate the apples in a separate bowl, and melt the margarine.

Spray a baking dish with cooking spray or rub with margarine. Spread a third of the dry mixture, cover with a third of the apples, repeating.

Pour melted margarine on top, and bake for 1 hour.

Banana Cheesecake

Ingredients

4 vegan wheat cookies

2 teaspoons vegetable oil, divided

2 (12 ounce) packages firm silken tofu

2 medium sized ripe bananas (not over ripe)

1/4 cup-1/2 cup brown sugar, to taste

1/4 cup nondairy milk

1 teaspoon ground cinnamon, optional

1 tablespoon vanilla

pinch sea salt

cinnamon, to taste, to garnish

brown sugar, to taste, to garnish

Directions

Preheat oven to 350 degrees F. In food processor or blender, pulverize cookies into a powder. Grease a 10x10" (at least 4" deep) glass or ceramic pan with 1 teaspoon of the oil. Coat pan with the cookie crumbs and pour the other teaspoon oil over the crumbs.

In food processor or blender, blend all of the other ingredients (except garnishes) until smooth, stopping to push it down the sides if necessary.

With a large spoon, ladle the filling over the cookie crumbs, being careful not to disturb them. Smooth over the top and sprinkle with the cinnamon and brown sugar.

Bake for 1 hour or until brown on edges. Remove and cool completely or refrigerate.

Coconut Lemon Cake

Ingredients

20 oz sugar

8 oz non-hydrogenated margarine

¼ cup lemon juice

grated zest of 4 lemons

2 teaspoons vanilla

1 ½ tablespoons lemon extract

24.6 oz flour

2 tablespoons baking powder

1 ½ teaspoons baking soda

1 ½ teaspoons salt

2 cups water

2 cups premium coconut milk

Filling

¾ - 1 cup pure raspberry jam, warmed slightly until spreadable

1/3 cup fine-shred coconut

Directions

Preheat oven to 350F, grease 2 9x13 pans.

Cream together sugar and margarine. Add lemon juice, zest, vanilla and lemon extracts and beat well. Whisk together dry ingredients in a medium bowl.

Add dry ingredients in three sections, alternating with the water and coconut milk. Beat well after each addition. Divide between pans and bake 45 minutes, or until cake tests done.

Cool completely in the pan before turning out onto a tray, then chill 1 hour before filling. Spread jam evenly over one of the layers and sprinkle with coconut.

Place second layer on top, trim the edges and chill again before frosting and decorating.

Chocolate Banana Cake

Ingredients

2 very ripe medium bananas

1 1/4 cups all-purpose white, unbleached flour

3/4 cup sugar (half white and half brown)

1/4 cup unsweetened cocoa powder

1/3 cup canola oil

1/3 cup water

1 teaspoon baking soda

1 teaspoon white vinegar

1/4 teaspoon salt

1/3 cup vegan semisweet chocolate chips

Directions

Preheat oven to 350F. Mash bananas or blend with electric beater.

Blend in wet ingredients and brown sugar. Sift dry ingredients together then add to wet.

Blend well then pour into a greased 8X8 square cake pan. Sprinkle chocolate chips over batter.

Bake about 35 minutes or until toothpick inserted in the center comes out clean. Cool completely before serving.

Creamy Peanut Butter Pie

Ingredients

Filling:

4 squares of unsweetened bakers chocolate

2/3 cup peanut butter

16-18oz silken tofu

1 cup sugar

4-6 tablespoon soy milk

Vegan graham cracker crust

Directions

Melt the chocolate and blend with the tofu, peanut butter, and sugar adding soy milk to the desired texture.

Pour filling into the graham cracker pie crust and refrigerate.

Raspberry Chocolate Cake

Ingredients

1 1/2 cups flour

1/3 cup unsweetened cacao powder

1/2 teaspoon baking soda

1/2 teaspoon sea salt

1 cup brown sugar

1/2 cup grapeseed oil

1 cup chilled brewed coffee

2 teaspoons vanilla extract

2 tablespoons apple cider vinegar

Chocolate Raspberry Frosting

2 ounces unsweetened dark chocolate

1/4 cup fresh raspberries, mashed

3 tablespoons water

1 teaspoon vanilla extract

1 cup confectioners' (icing) sugar

Topping over frosting

1 cup fresh raspberries

½ cup non-dairy chocolate chips

Directions

Preheat oven to 375°F. Spread coconut oil on baking dish to prevent sticking.

Sift flour, cacao, baking soda, salt and sugar. In another bowl, combine oil, coffee and vanilla. Pour liquid into dry, and mix until smooth.

Add vinegar and stir briefly; baking soda will begin to react with vinegar. Quickly pour batter into prepared pan.

Bake for 25 to 30 minutes. Allow cake to cool slightly before adding frosting.

Frosting:

In heavy saucepan, melt chocolate over low to medium heat. Once fully melted, remove from heat and stir in mashed raspberries, water and vanilla. Stir in confectioners' sugar. Spread frosting on cooled cake.

Top frosting with whole raspberries and sprinkle non-dairy chocolate chips over cake.

Pecan Cheesecake

Ingredients

Crust:

1/4 cup pecans (chopped)

3 tablespoon raw sugar

1 1/2 cup vanilla wafers or vegan graham crackers

1/4 cup margarine (melted)

Filling:

1 pound vegan cream cheese

1 1/4 cup sugar

2 tablespoon pastry flour

3 tablespoon applesauce

1 1/2 teaspoon vanilla

1/2 cup pecans (chopped)

Directions

Crust:

Blend all ingredients except margarine. In mixing bowl, add wafer mixture and melted margarine to moisten. Place mixture in round foil pie pan, pressing down to cover the whole pan.

Bake at 350 F for 6 minutes. Remove from oven.

Filling:

Mix vegan cream cheese and sugar in bowl. Stir in flour, slowly add applesauce. Stir in vanilla and pecans.

Mix all ingredients well. Pour mixture onto wafer crust and bake at 350 F for 1 hour. Garnish top of cheesecake with pecan halves.

Vanilla Cake

Ingredients

1 1/2 cups flour

1 cup sugar

1/2 teaspoon baking soda

1/2 teaspoon salt

1 cup ice cold water

1/2 cup oil

2 teaspoons vanilla

2 tablespoons lemon juice

Directions

Preheat oven to 375 F. Grease an 8" or 9" cake pan. In a bowl, sift together flour, sugar, baking soda and salt until very fine.

In a small bowl, combine cold water, oil, and vanilla. Add liquid ingredients (except lemon juice) to dry and combine. Once the batter is combined, add the lemon juice and stir quickly then pour into prepared pan.

Bake for 25 to 30 minutes or until toothpick comes out clean.

Carrot Cake

Ingredients

1 1/2 cup self rising flour

1 cup raw sugar

1 teaspoon baking soda

1 teaspoon cinnamon

1/4 teaspoon salt

1 cup of shredded carrots

3/4 cup orange juice

1/3 cup grapeseed oil

1 teaspoon vanilla

1 tablespoon ground flax seed

Directions

Heat oven to 350F. Mix all dry ingredients in bowl. then add carrots. Stir until well coated. Add remaining wet ingredients and stir just until blended. Pour into ungreased 9 inch square non stick pan.

Bake 25-30 minutes. Let cool before serving.

Spice Cake

Ingredients

3 cups flour

2 cups sugar

2 bags of chai tea

2 teaspoons baking soda

1 teaspoon salt

2 cups water

1/3 cup olive or vegetable oil

2 teaspoons vanilla

2 teaspoons cinnamon

2 tablespoons vinegar

Directions

Preheat oven to 350F.

Cut open the bags of chai tea and pour out the spices. In a bowl add the dry ingredients together and stir. Then add the water, oil and vanilla. Add the vinegar in last mixing in well, and pour mixture into cake pan.

Bake at 350F for 40 minute to an hour, or until toothpick comes out clean.

Cranberry Banana Cookies

Ingredients

1 banana

1 cup soft margarine

1/2 cup white sugar

1/2 cup packed brown sugar

1 teaspoon vanilla

1.5 cups flour

1 teaspoon baking soda

1 teaspoon cinnamon

1 teaspoon ground nutmeg

3 cups oatmeal

1/2 cup dried cranberries

1/2 cup sliced almonds

Directions

Preheat over to 350F. Mash banana with a fork, then mix with margarine, sugars, and vanilla in a bowl until smooth.

In a separate bowl, mix the flour, baking soda, cinnamon, and nutmeg. Mix the wet with the dry, then add oatmeal, cranberries, and almonds.

Spoon onto a ungreased cookie sheet, and bake for about 15 minutes. Let cool and serve.

Chocolate Chip Cookies

Ingredients

2 cups all purpose flour

2 teaspoons baking powder

1/2 teaspoons sea salt

2 teaspoons cinnamon

1 cup sugar

1/2 cup canola oil

1 teaspoons vanilla

1/2 cup water

1 cup vegan chocolate chips

Directions

Preheat oven to 350 F.

Mix all ingredients together in a large bowl, until well combined.

Using a small scoop, place mixture on a lightly greased cookie sheet.

Bake 10-12 minutes. (Note: Cookies won't brown on top when done.)

Gingersnap Cookies

Ingredients

4 tablespoons margarine

1/2 cup raw sugar

Egg replacer equivalent to 1 egg

2 1/2 cups plain flour

1 teaspoon bicarbonate of soda

4 teaspoon ground ginger

1 teaspoon ground cloves

2 teaspoon ground cinnamon

2 teaspoon ground nutmeg

3 tablespoons golden syrup

Directions

Preheat oven to 350F.

Cream margarine and raw sugar, add egg replacement, mix. Add flour, soda and spices, then golden syrup and mix well.

Roll mixture into teaspoon sized balls, flatten slightly and place on cookie tray.

Bake for 10 minutes in at 350F.

Green Tea Cookies

Ingredients

½ cup vegan butter spread

½ cup unrefined coconut oil (not refined)

2 tablespoons matcha green tea powder

¼ cup + ½ cup powdered sugar, divided

¼ cup sweetened shredded coconut (optional)

2¼ cups all-purpose flour

Directions

Preheat oven to 400º F.

Cream together buttery spread, coconut oil, green tea powder and ¼ cup powdered sugar until smooth. Add shredded coconut and flour and mix until combined. Mixture will be somewhat crumbly but should stick together.

Roll dough into 24 balls, approximately 1½ inches in size. Place on an ungreased cookie sheet and bake in preheated oven for 10-12 minutes or just until set.

Place ½ cup powdered sugar in a wide, shallow dish; set aside.

Remove cookies from oven and allow to cool for 10-15 minutes. Roll each cookie in powdered sugar and set aside until completely cooled.

Peanut Butter Balls

Ingredients

3/4 cup raw pumpkin seeds

3/4 cup raw sunflower seeds

1/2 cup pitted dates

1/2 cup peanut butter

1 tablespoon chia seeds

Directions

Blend together all ingredients, using a food processor.

Roll into balls and chill in refrigerator.

Raisin Cookies

Ingredients

1 1/2 cups firmly packed brown sugar

1 cup margarine

Egg replacer equivalent to 2 eggs

2 teaspoons water

2 teaspoons vanilla extract

2 cups all purpose flour

1 teaspoon baking powder

1 teaspoon baking soda

2 teaspoons ground cinnamon

1/2 teaspoon salt

2 cups quick-cooking oats, uncooked

1 cup raisins

Directions

Preheat oven to 350 F. Combine brown sugar and margarine in bowl and mix with spoon. Add egg replacer, water and vanilla, and continue mixing.

Add all remaining ingredients except oats and raisins. Mix well. Stir in oats and raisins.

Drop dough by rounded tablespoonfuls, 2 inches apart, onto cookie sheets. Bake 9-

11 minutes or until lightly browned. Let stand 1 minute. Remove from cookie sheets, cool completely before serving.

Chocolate Chip Pumpkin Cookies

Ingredients

1 cup vegetable oil

4 cup sugar

2 egg substitute (flax seeds and water works well)

5 cups flour

1/4 teaspoon ground ginger

2 teaspoons baking powder

2 teaspoons baking soda

2 teaspoons nutmeg

2 teaspoons cinnamon

1 teaspoon all-spice

1 3/4 teaspoons salt

1 29 oz. can of pumpkin

2 cup vegan chocolate chips

1 cup chopped walnuts

Directions

Beat oil and vegan sugar in mixing bowl. Add egg substitutes and beat well.

In a separate bowl, stir together the flour, baking powder, baking soda, spices, and salt.

Add vegan sugar mixture alternatively with pumpkin into flour mixture. Stir well after each addition. Fold in chocolate chips, walnuts, and vanilla.

Drop by teaspoon onto a greased cookie sheet. Bake for 15-20 minutes or until golden brown at 350 F.

Peanut Butter Cookies

Ingredients

3 tablespoons egg replacer + 4 tablespoons water

2 1/4 cups unbleached whole wheat flour

1 1/4 cup natural crunchy peanut butter

2/3 cup maple syrup

1/2 cup Sucanat

1/2 cup margarine

1/2 tablespoon baking powder

Directions

Preheat oven to 350 F. Mix egg replacer and water. In large bowl, combine all ingredients, and mix.

Roll tablespoons of dough into balls, and place 2" apart on cookie sheet. Flatten balls with flour dipped fork, in criss-cross pattern.

Bake 15 minutes or until lightly browned.

About the Author

Brad Cox is author of several cookbooks on Vegan diet. He has written research papers on the topic and currently lives in California.